Suzie Dedications

- **Nicholas Kelly**

    - **Thank you, to my friends, family, and all the people who assisted in making this book a reality. This book is extremely personal, as it represents a promise I made to myself, because of the people I've lost. The idea to write a CF centered children's book was inspired by my late "Cyster" Michele Held (Shelly) and my "Fibro" Nicholas Statford (Vincent – evil snicker). Writing a CF book was a dream of theirs to complete together. However, since both have past, I knew I needed to make our dream a reality. Thus, this is for them, the CF community, and all the ones lost. #BreatheEasy**

- **Maria Rohan**

    - **"To all the patients I've loved like my own, who have died taking a piece of me with them. Breathe Easy, my loves. Your struggle and sacrifice has inspired me to work constantly for a better day in medicine. To St. Xenia and St. John Maximovitch I thank you, for guiding, protecting and through your intercession, having mercy on me.**

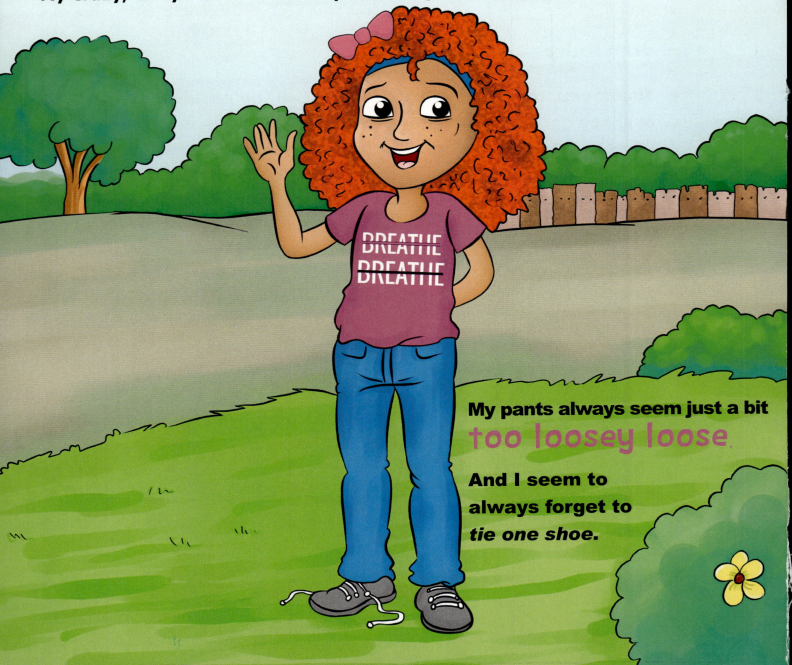

Hello! Hello! Hello to you.

I'm Miss Messy Suzie McGoo.
My crazy, curly red hair is always a messy-bobba-de-do.

My pants always seem just a bit *too loosey loose*.

And I seem to always forget to *tie one shoe.*

But I have Cystic Fibrosis lungs, just like you, and I cannot leave my lungs messy, no matter what I do!

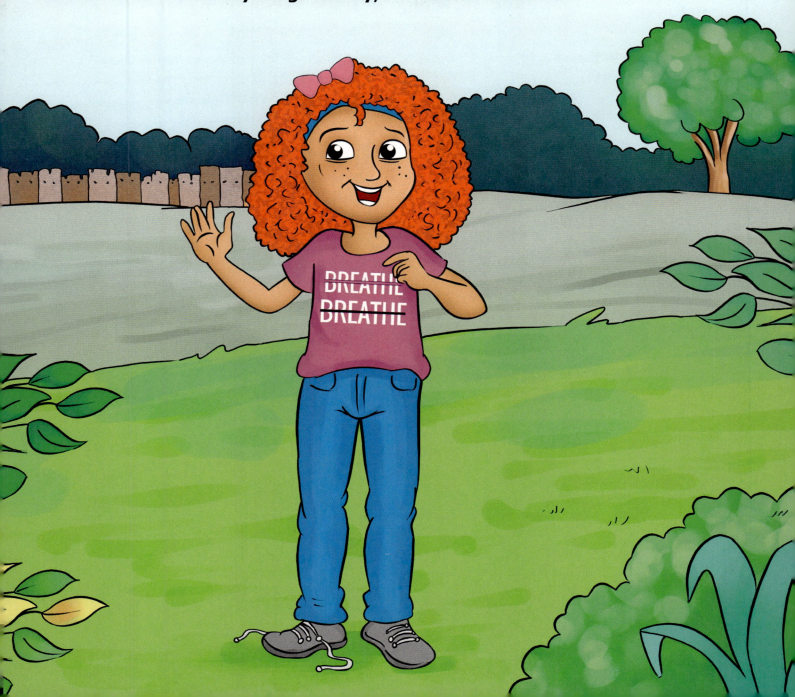

I eat all my fruits and veggies so I can get big and strong and grow high into the sky.

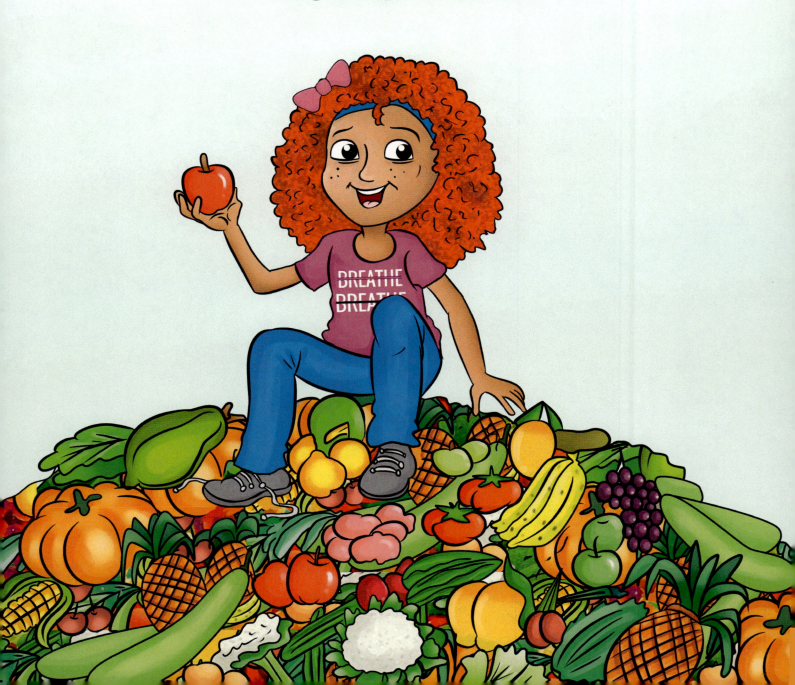

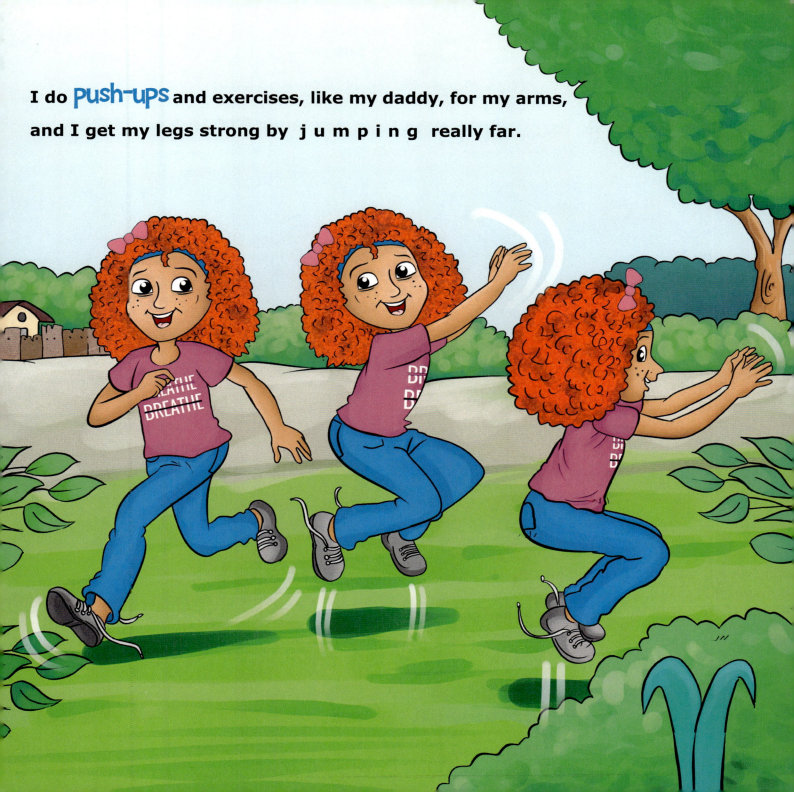

I do push-ups and exercises, like my daddy, for my arms, and I get my legs strong by j u m p i n g really far.

But we, but we,

Miss Messy Suzie McGoo and you,

have to do extra exercises to keep our lungs **strong** and **new**.

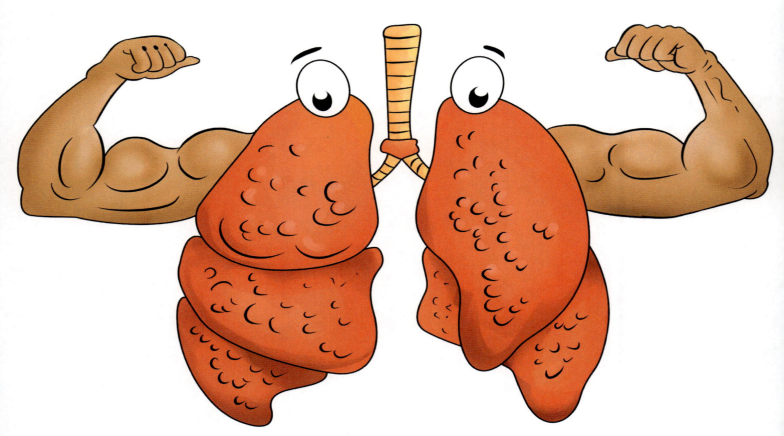

Ooo, ooo, ooo,

Hippity dippity doo!

Now that I've met you,

I have a big secret to tell you!

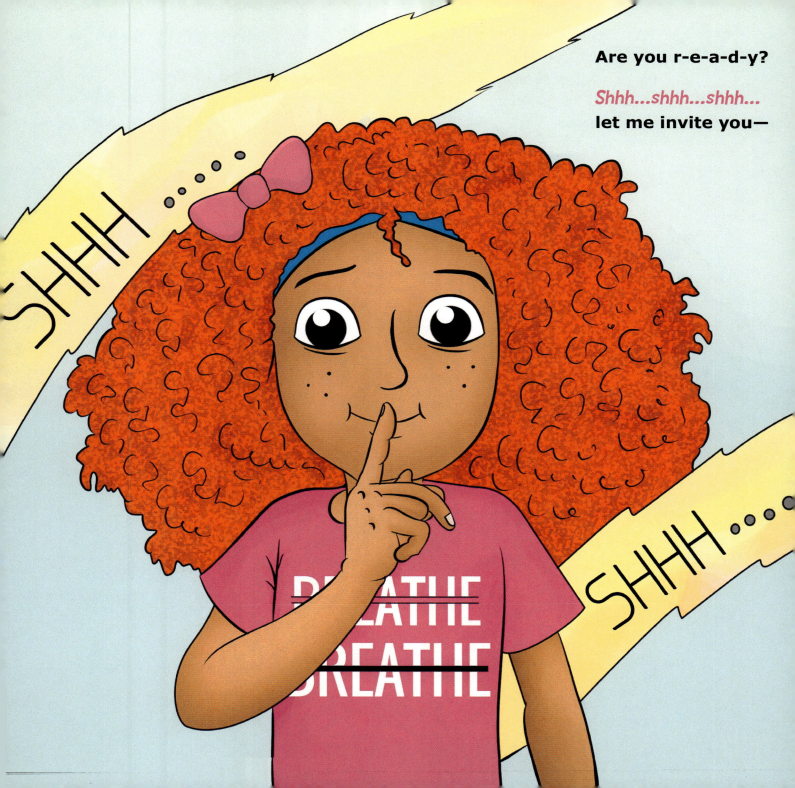

to the Miss Messy Suzie McGoo Secret Cuff Cough Crew.

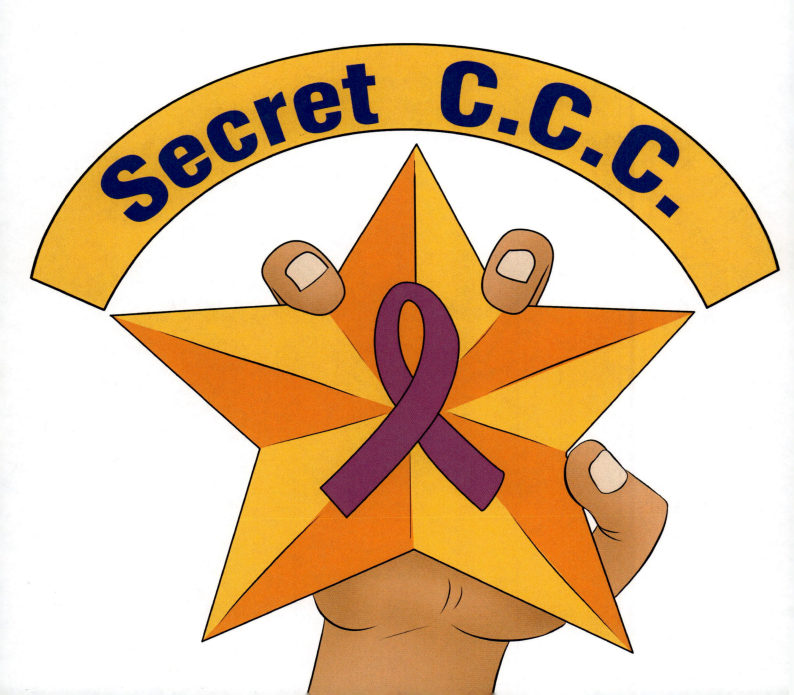

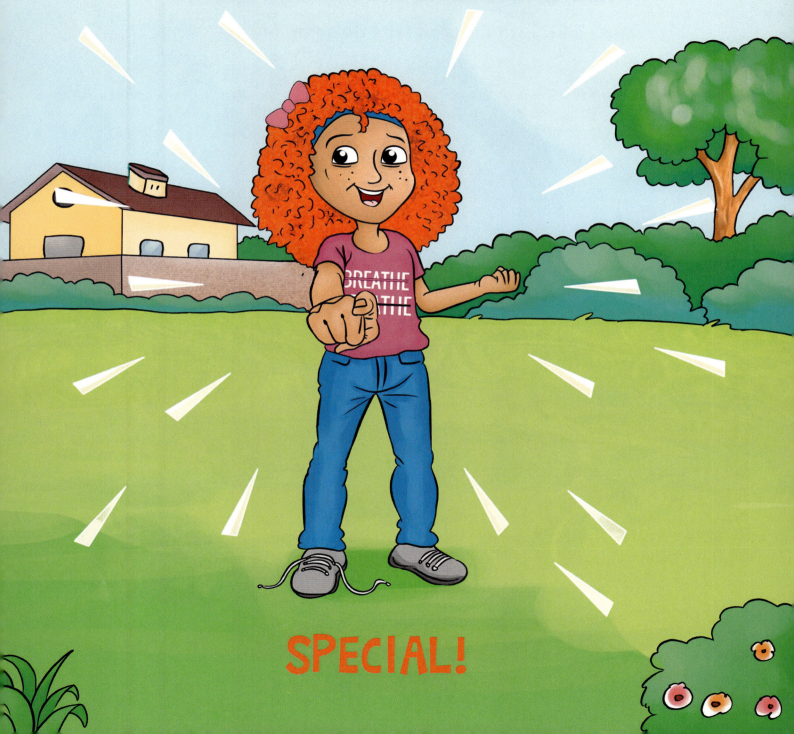

It's only for special CFers just like me and you!

SPECIAL!

Now, use your **ears** and **listen** carefully,
and come with me, and let's do some lung therapy!

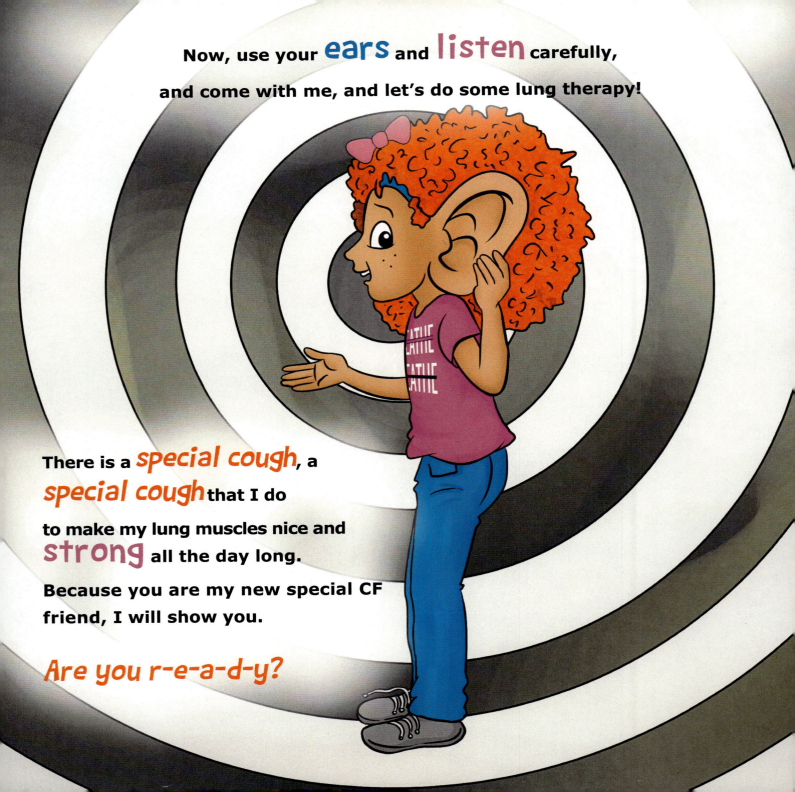

There is a *special cough*, a *special cough* that I do to make my lung muscles nice and **strong** all the day long.

Because you are my new special CF friend, I will show you.

Are you r-e-a-d-y?

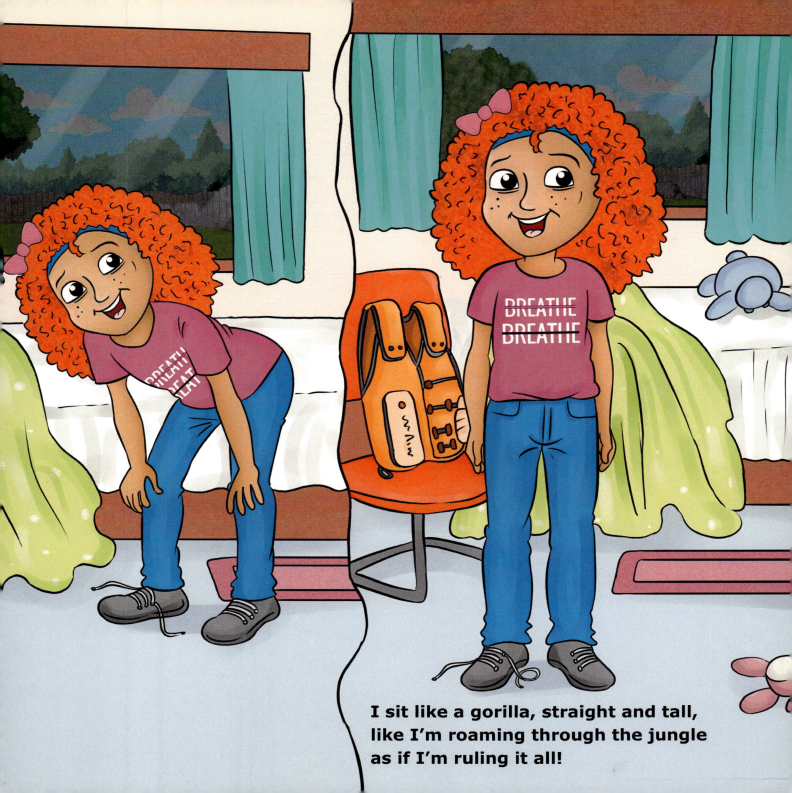
I sit like a gorilla, straight and tall, like I'm roaming through the jungle as if I'm ruling it all!

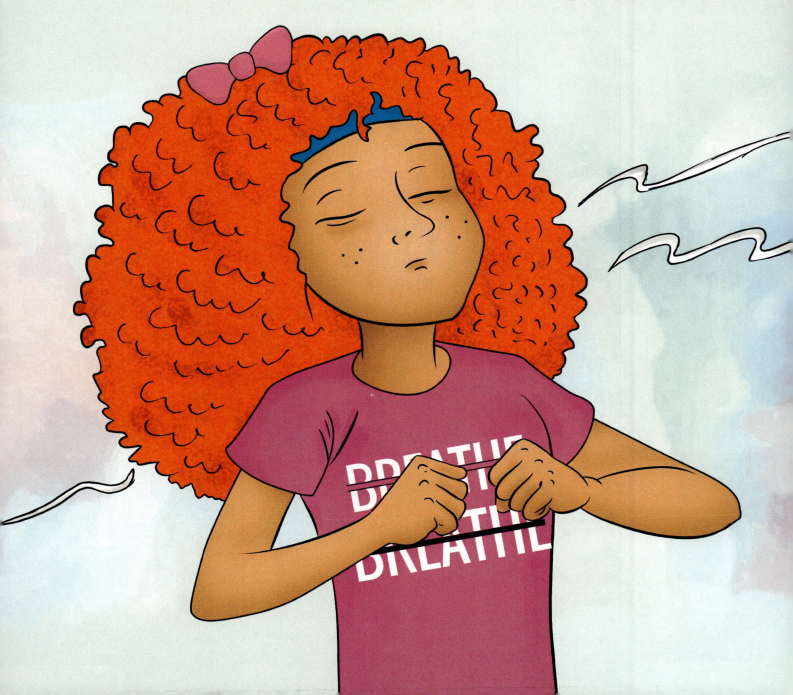

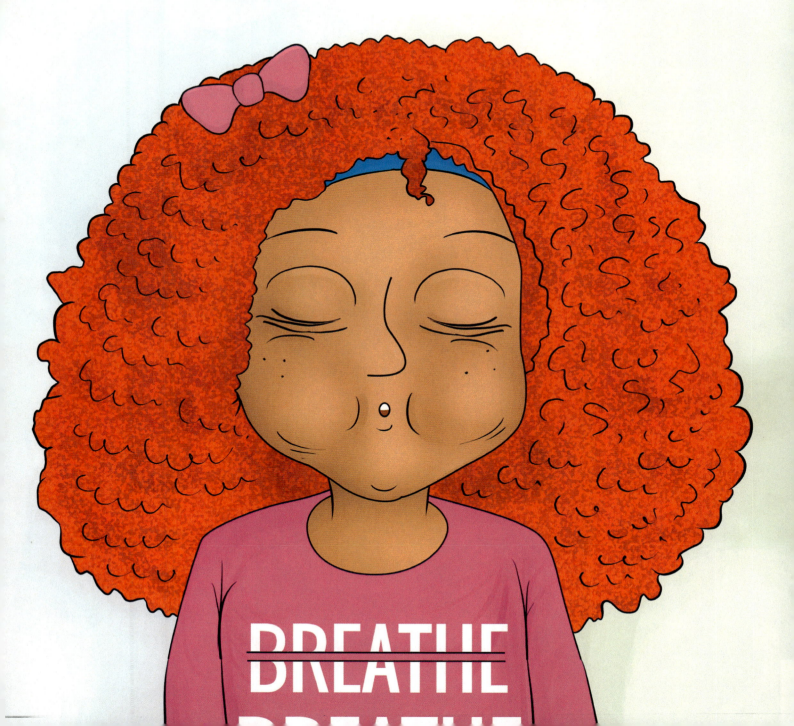

and f-r-e-e-e-e-z-e! Hold it for a second.

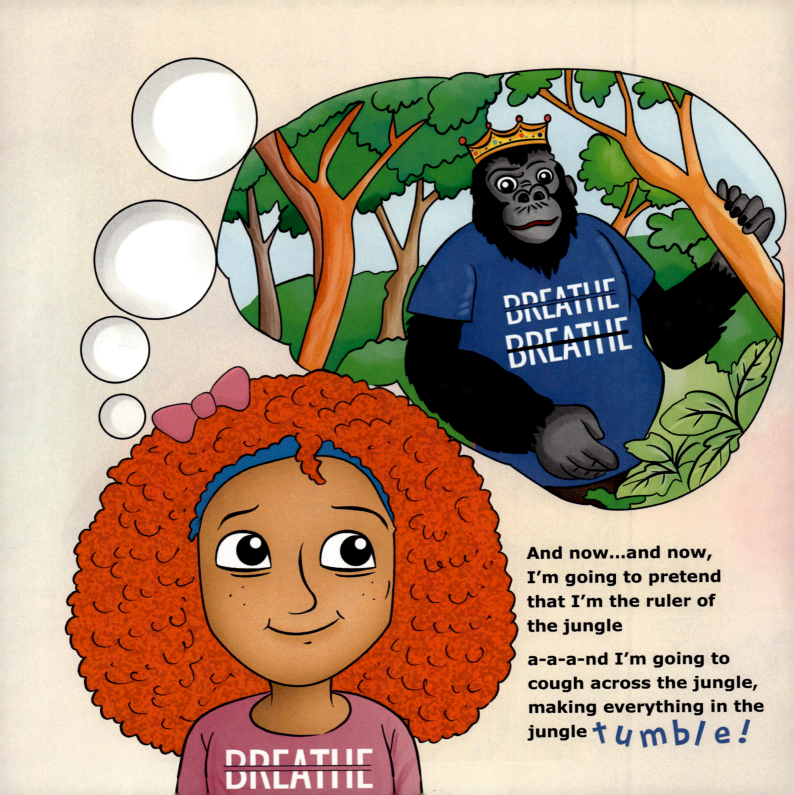

And now...and now, I'm going to pretend that I'm the ruler of the jungle

a-a-a-nd I'm going to cough across the jungle, making everything in the jungle tumble!

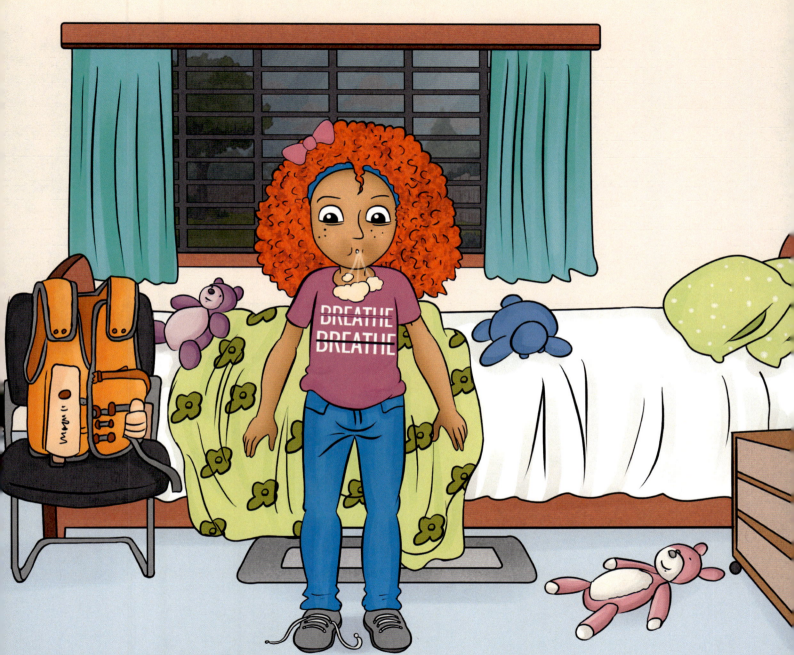

So I take a deep breath in,

and I'm going to bl-o-o-o-w the air out.

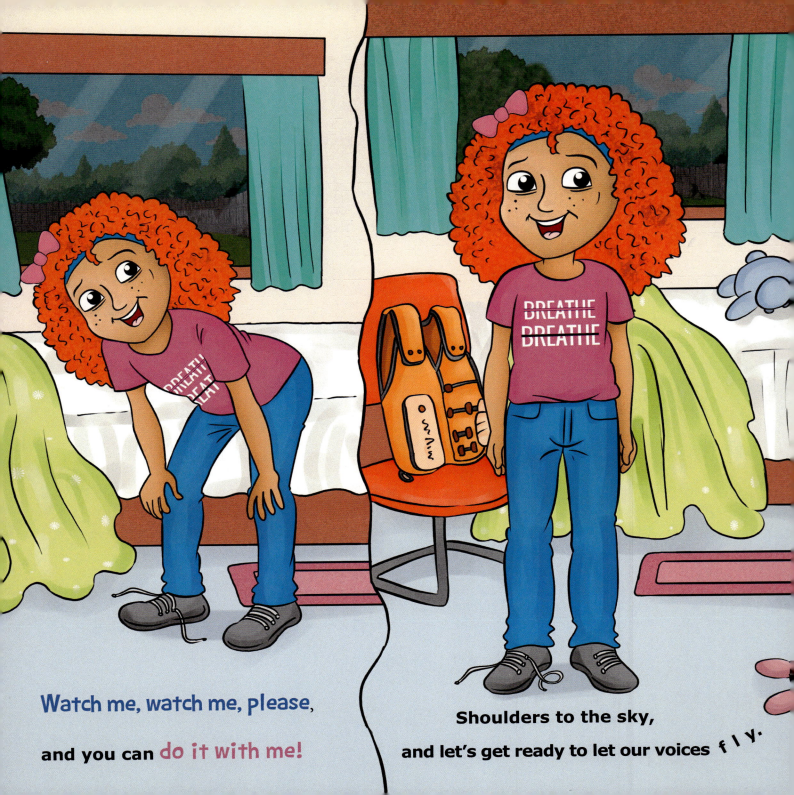

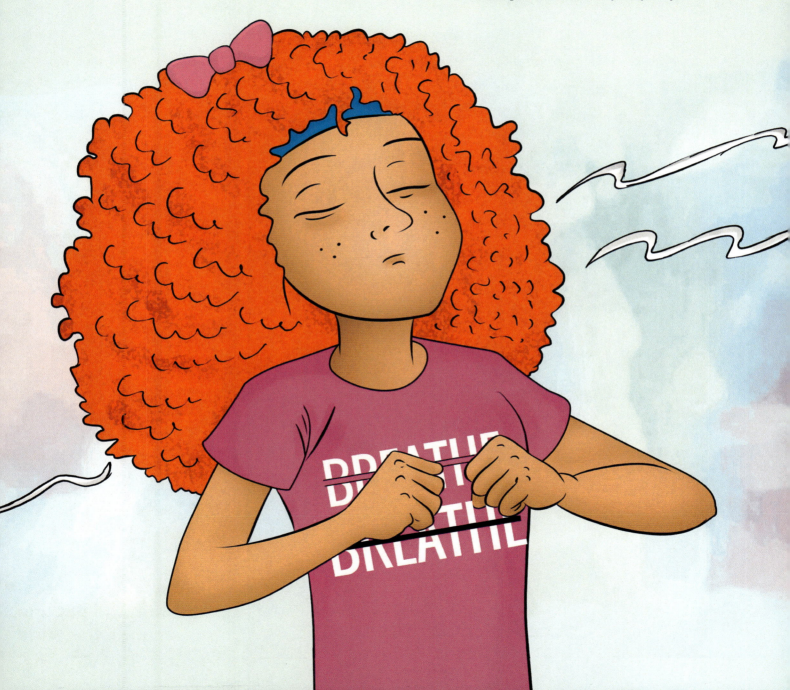

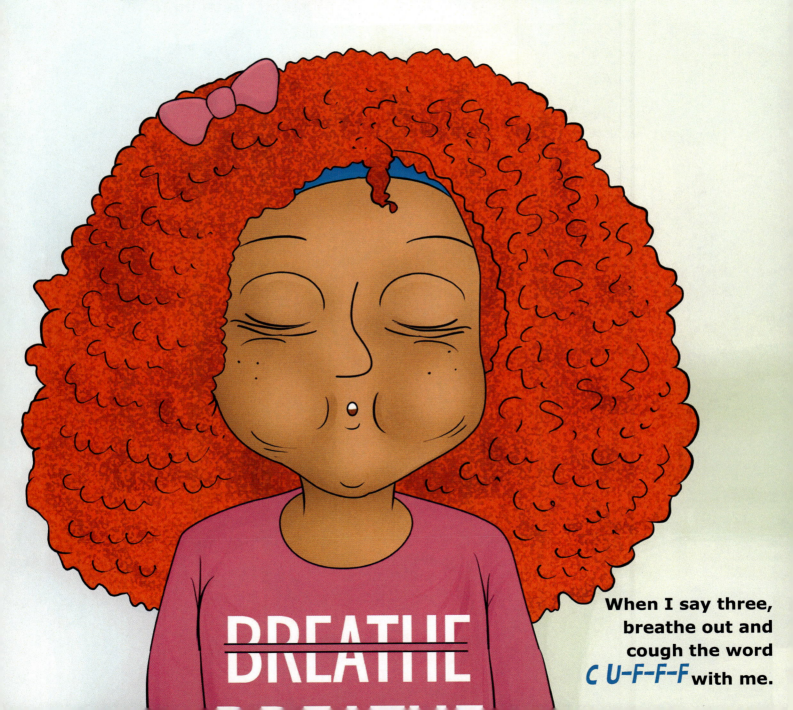

and f-r-e-e-e-e-z-e! Hold it for a second.

When I say three, breathe out and cough the word C U-F-F-F with me.

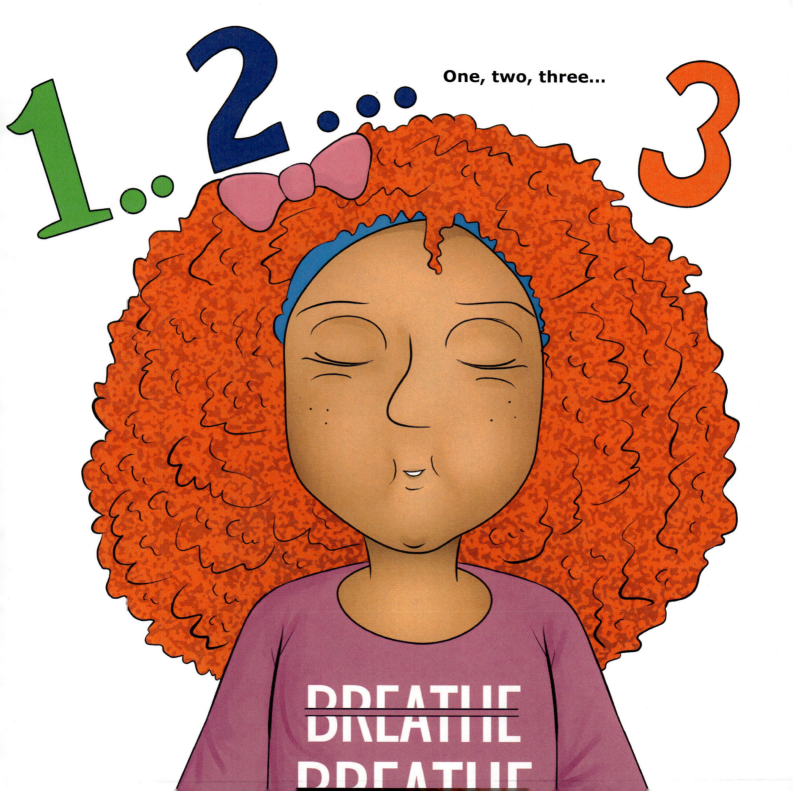

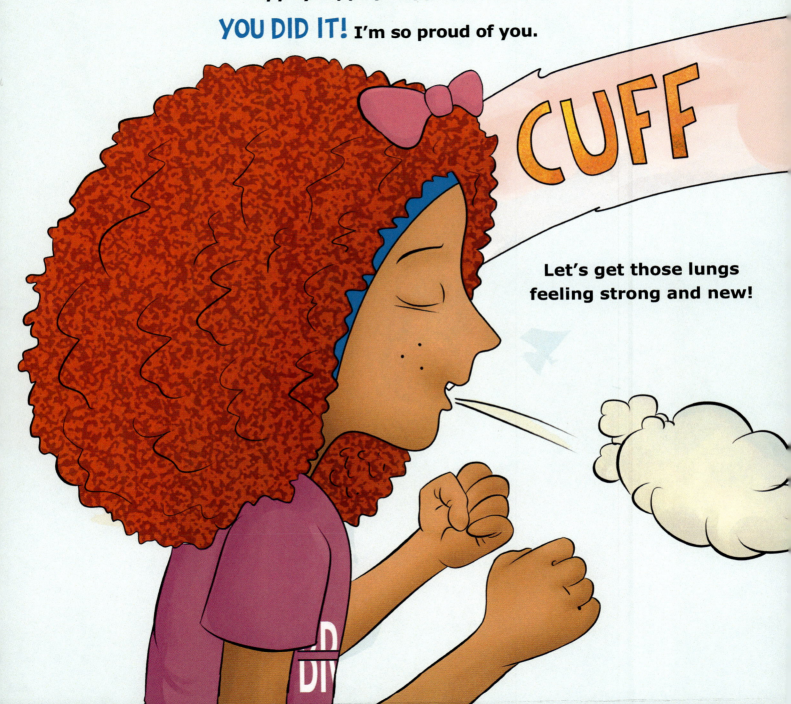

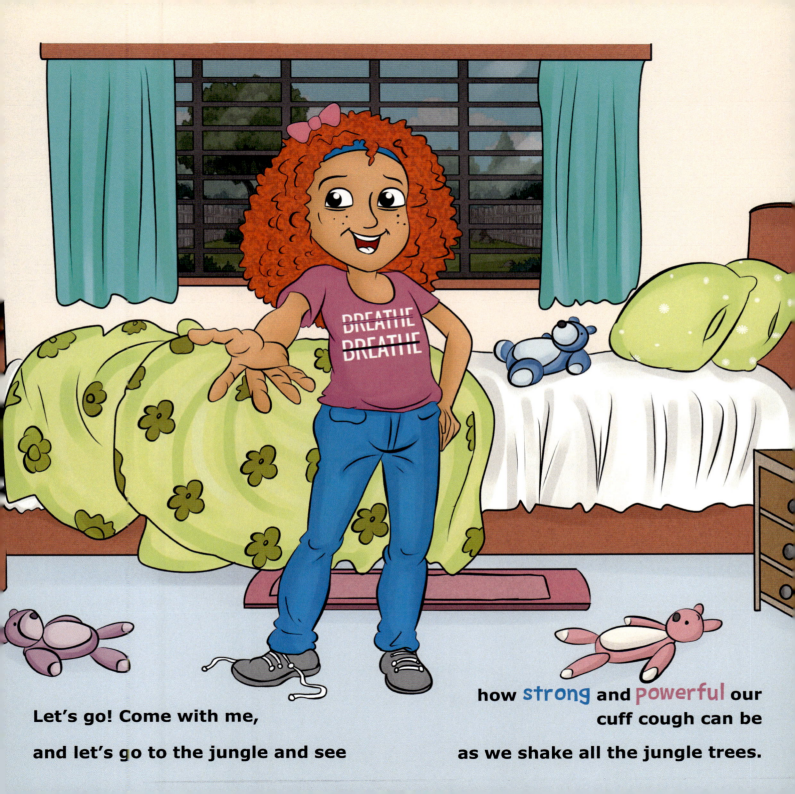

Let's go! Come with me,

and let's go to the jungle and see

how **strong** and **powerful** our cuff cough can be

as we shake all the jungle trees.

Close your eyes, and *hippity dippity kalamazoo!*

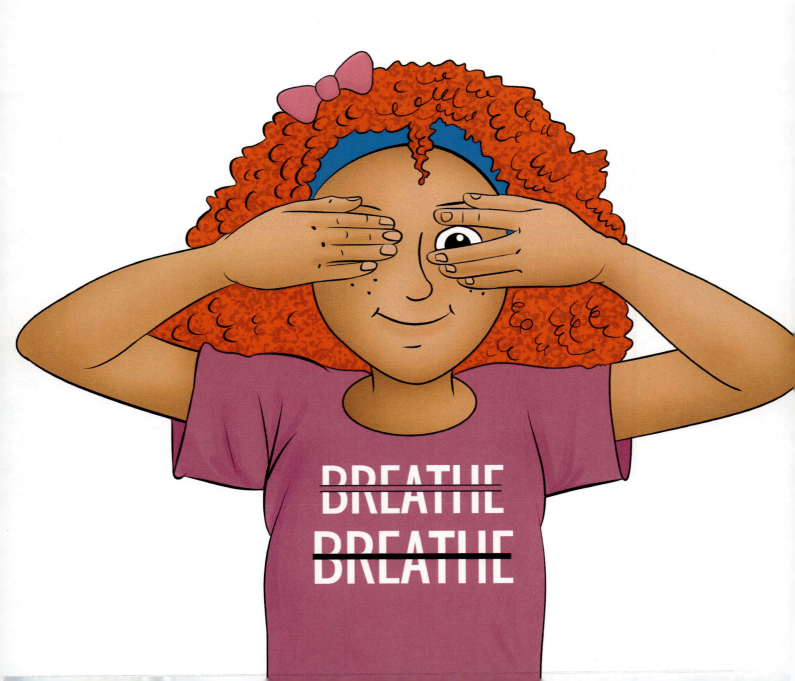

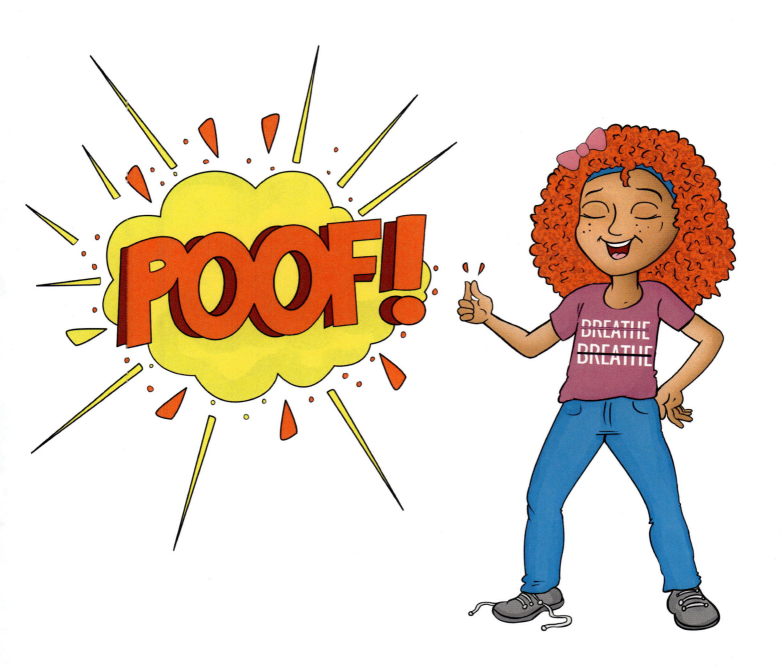

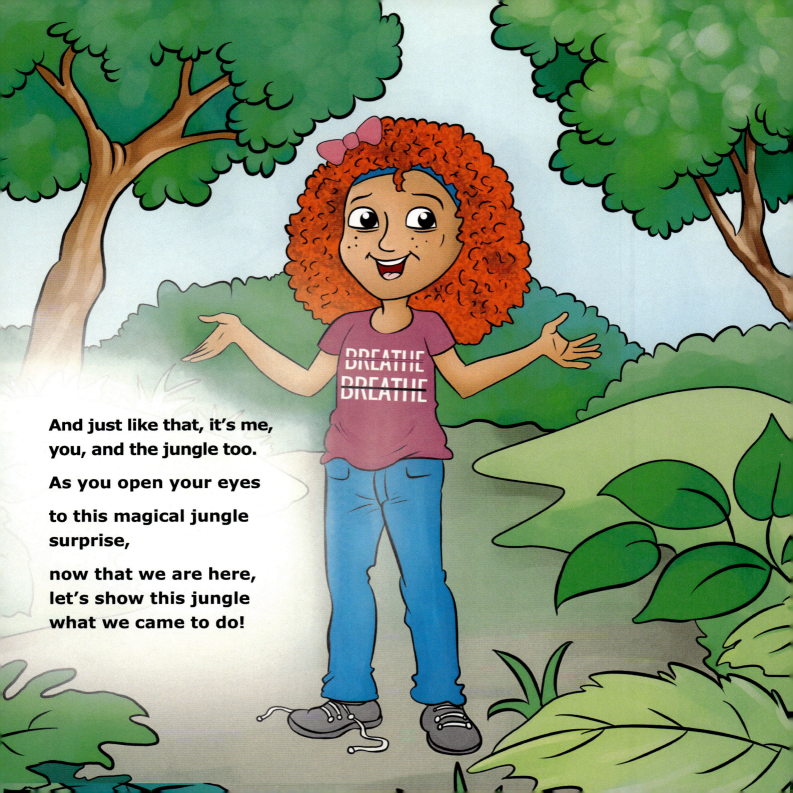

And just like that, it's me, you, and the jungle too.

As you open your eyes

to this magical jungle surprise,

now that we are here, let's show this jungle what we came to do!

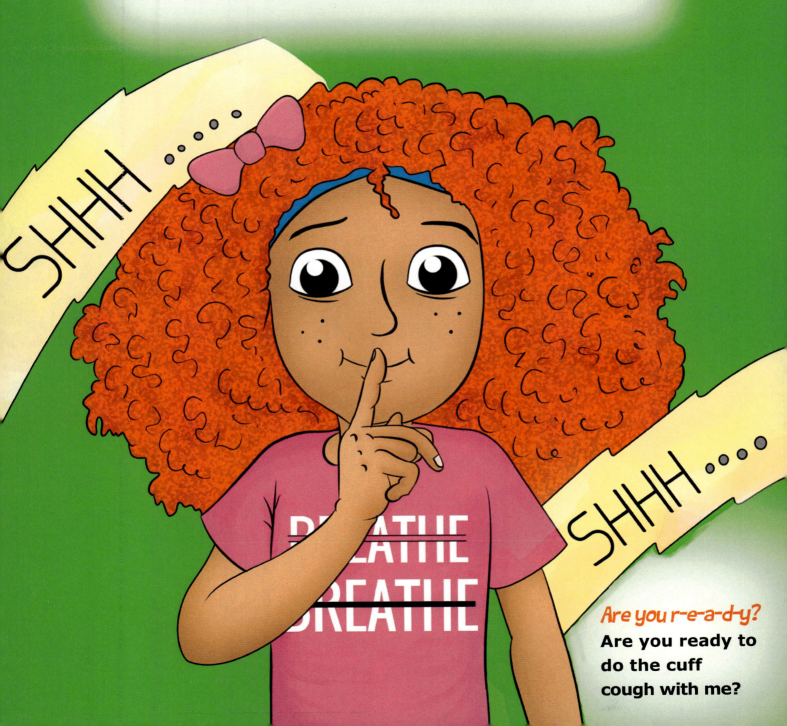

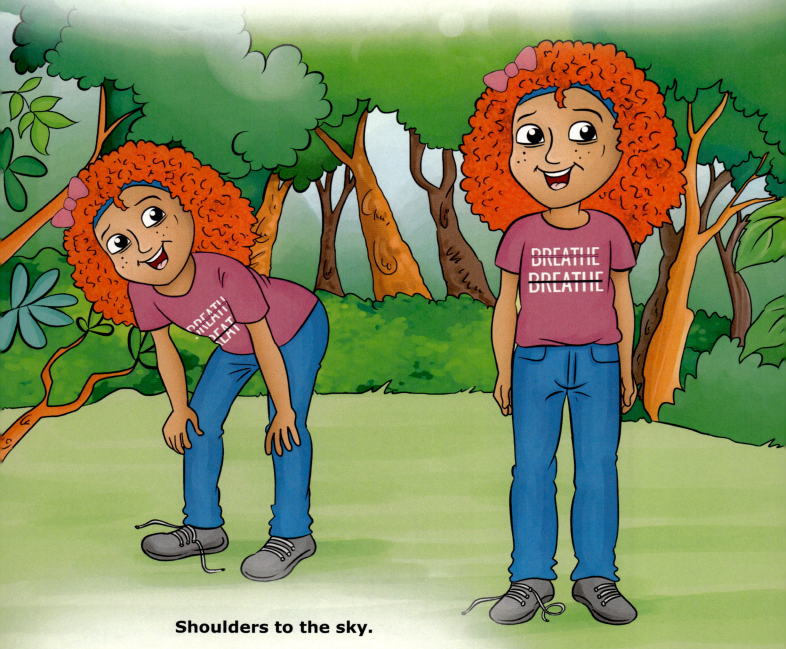

A-a-a-l-l-l righty, stand tall, like a gorilla in the jungle, ruling it all.

Shoulders to the sky.

And let's get ready to let our voices fly.

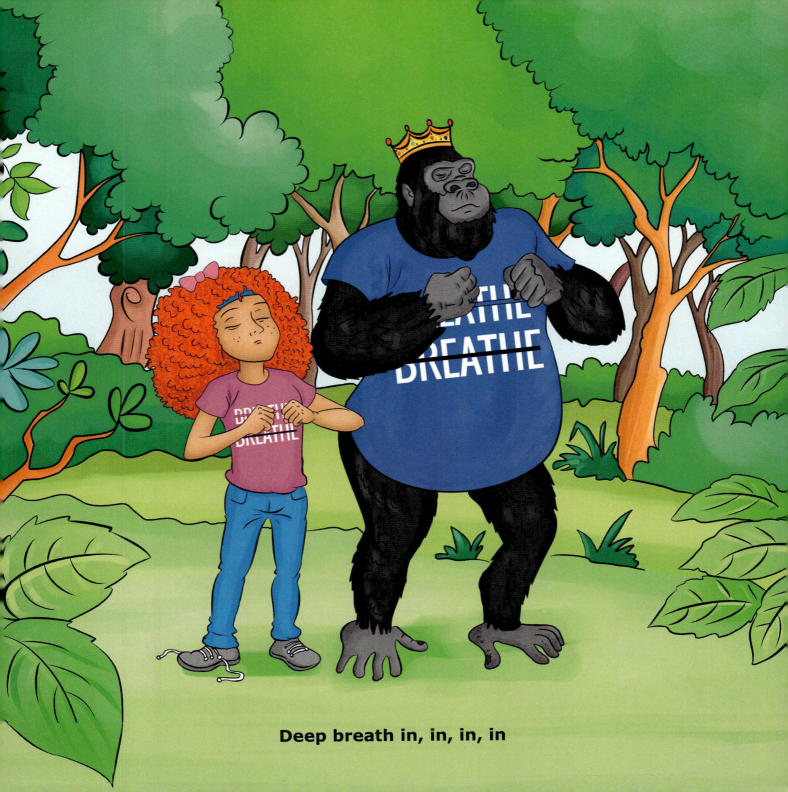
Deep breath in, in, in, in

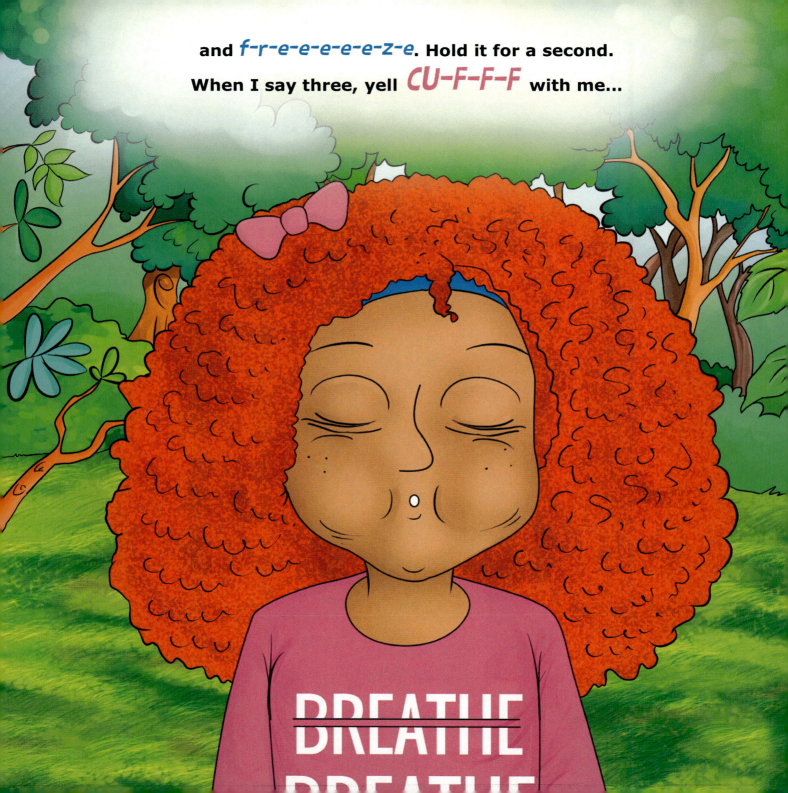

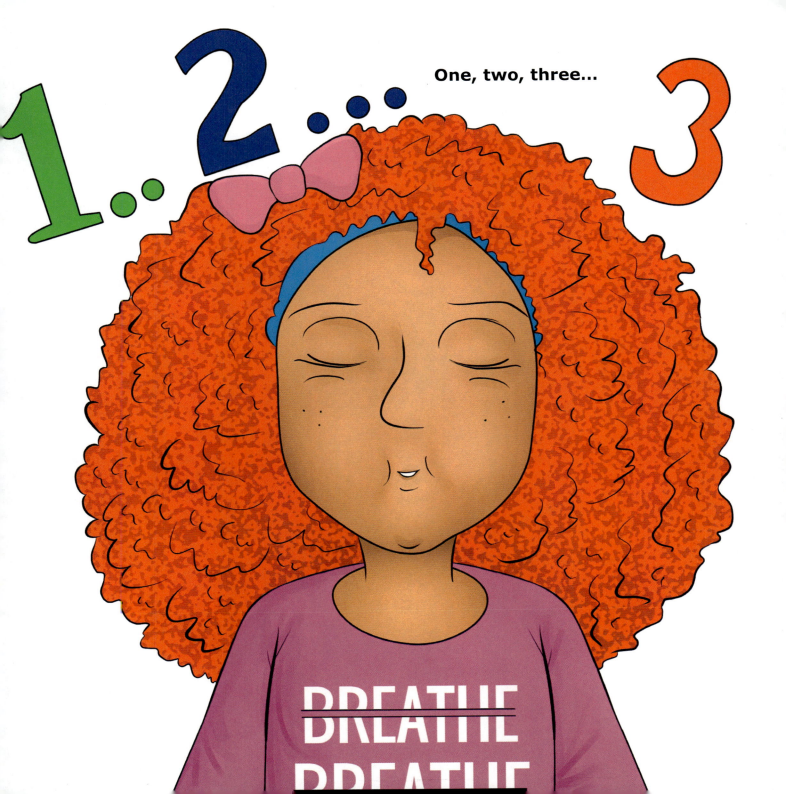

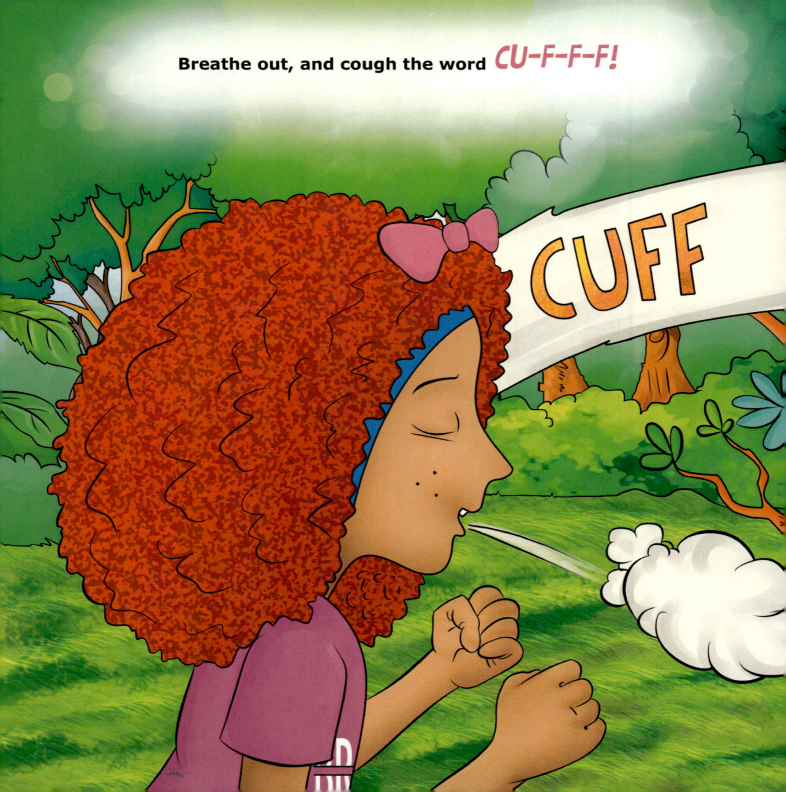

Hippity dippity doppity dee!

Did you see? Did you see?

Your **strong, powerful** cough made all the trees shake, even the leaves!

Again, again, my special CF friend, let's try it again with me.

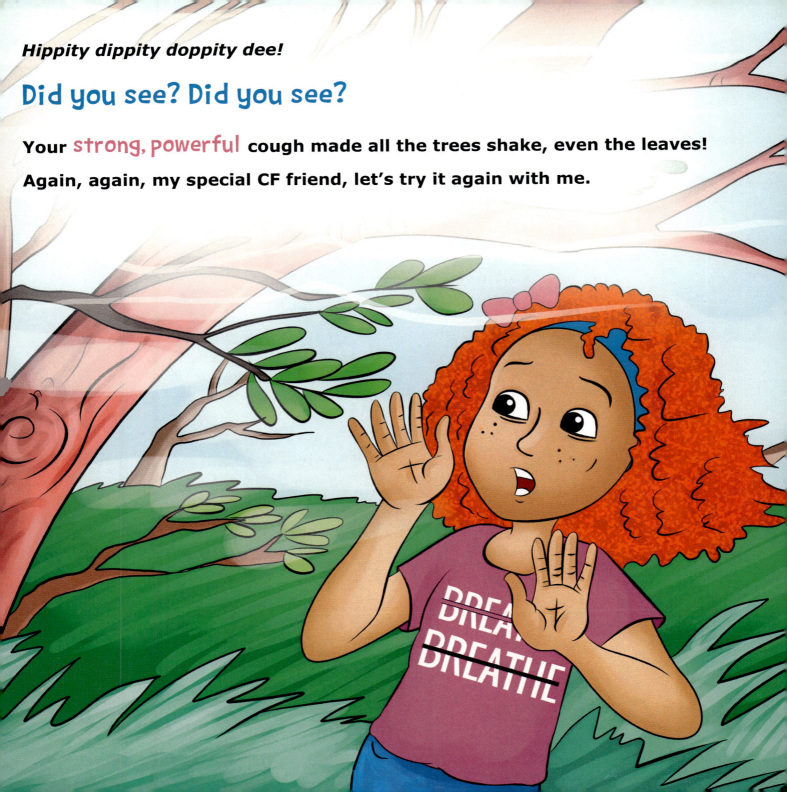

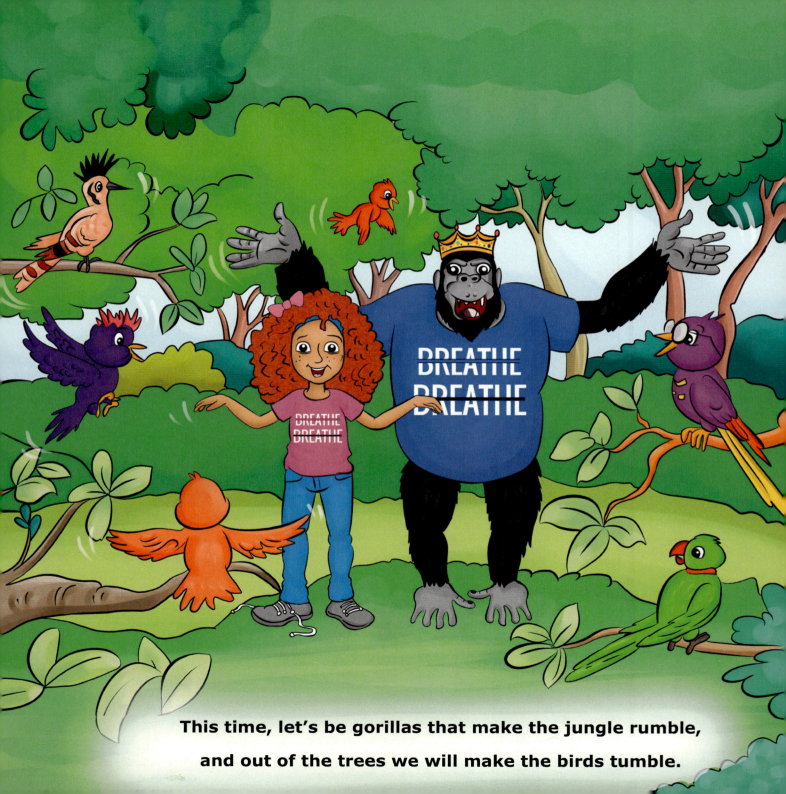

This time, let's be gorillas that make the jungle rumble, and out of the trees we will make the birds tumble.

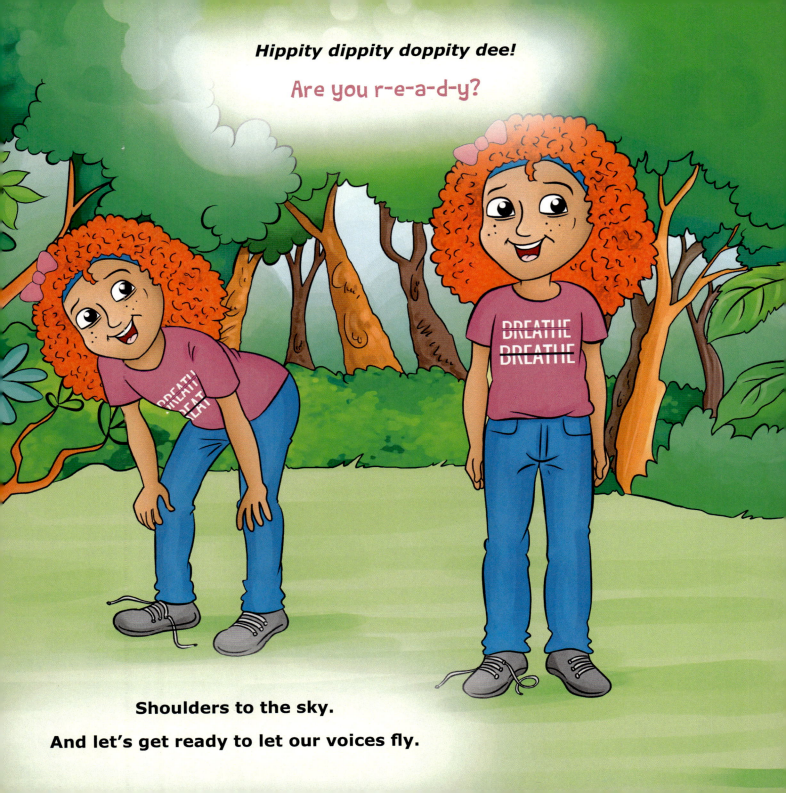

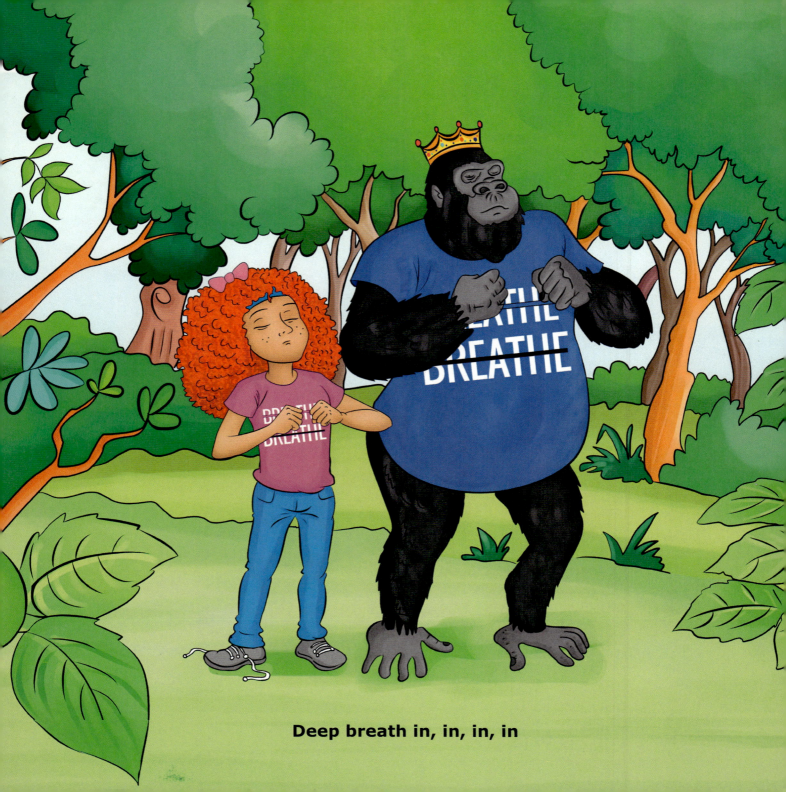
Deep breath in, in, in, in

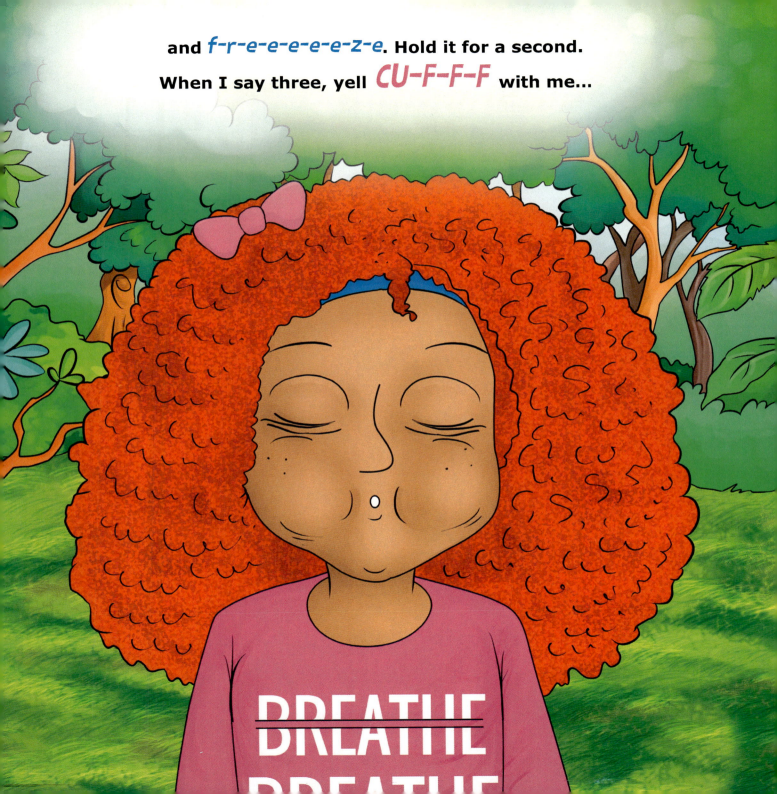

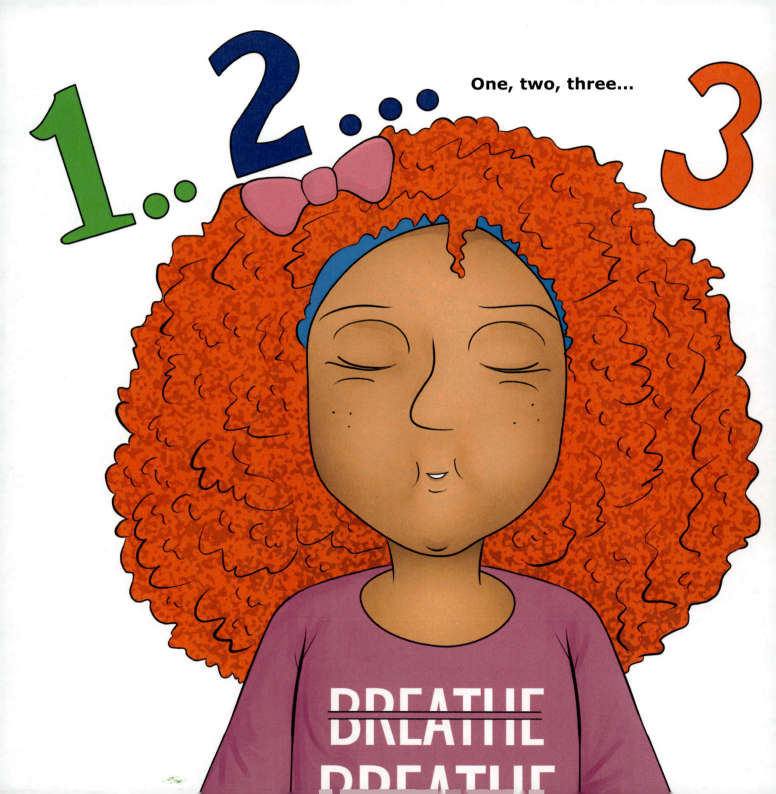

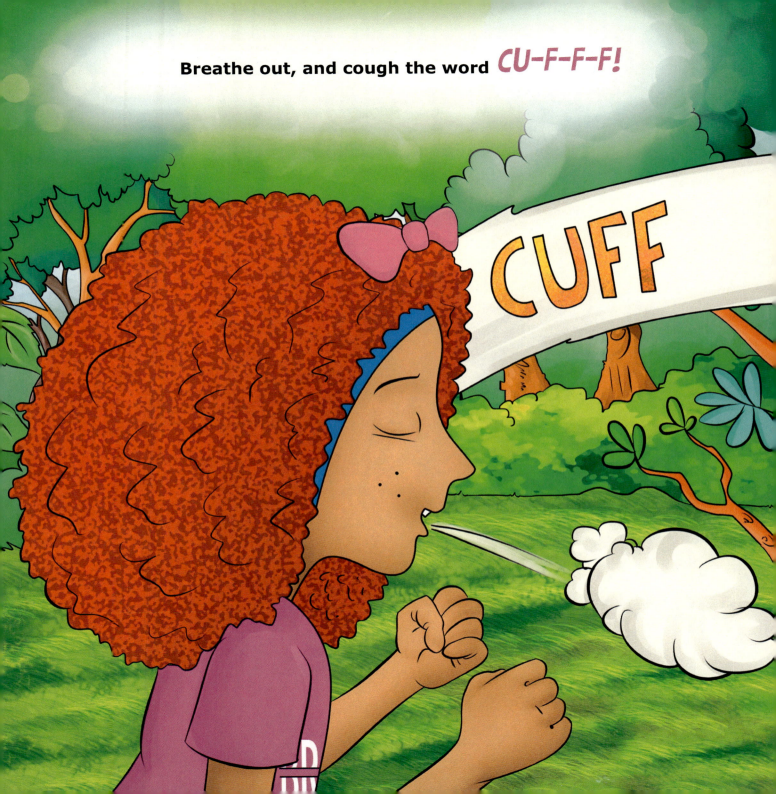

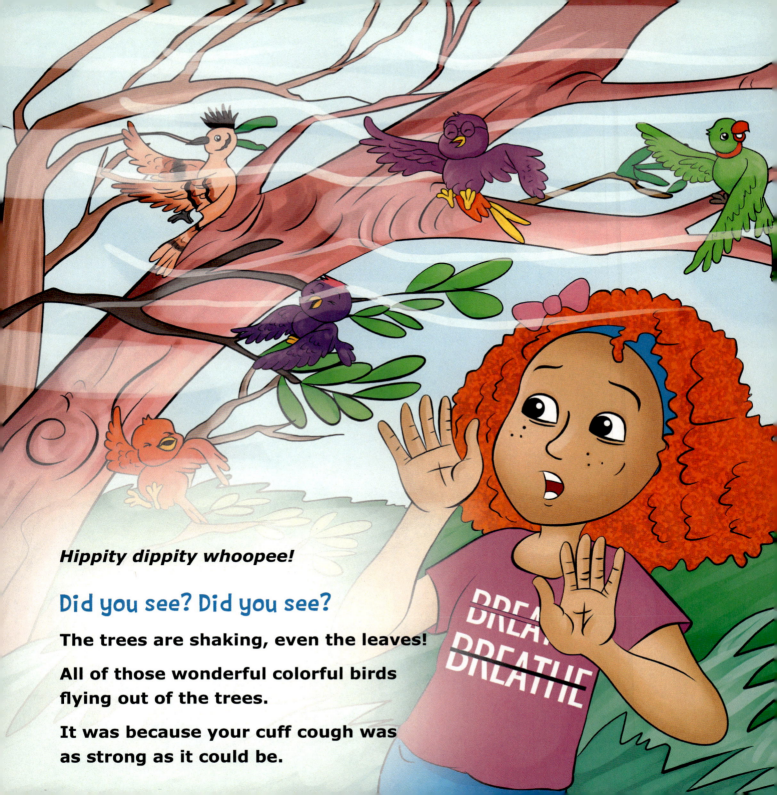

Hippity dippity whoopee!

Did you see? Did you see?

The trees are shaking, even the leaves!

All of those wonderful colorful birds flying out of the trees.

It was because your cuff cough was as strong as it could be.

I think, I think it's time to go home

before your momma notices you're gone.

Close your eyes, and *hippity dippity kalamazo!*

Back home, we go!

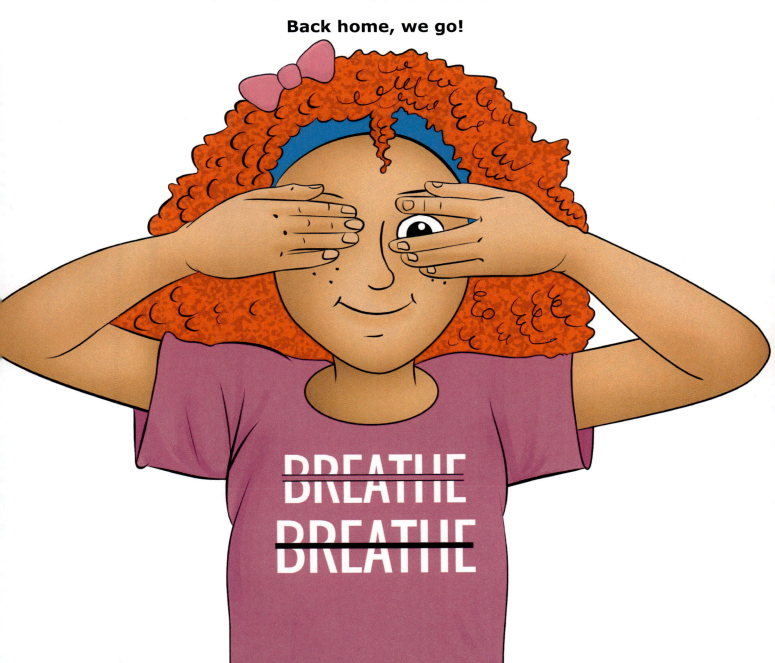

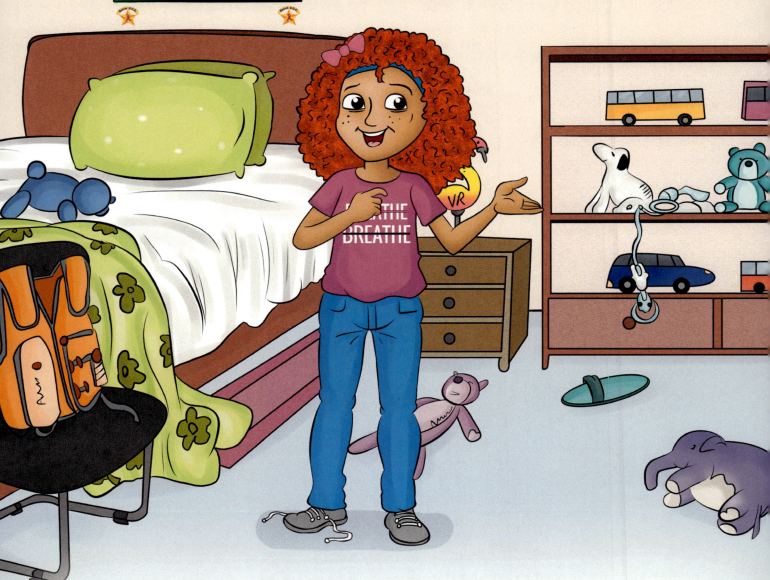

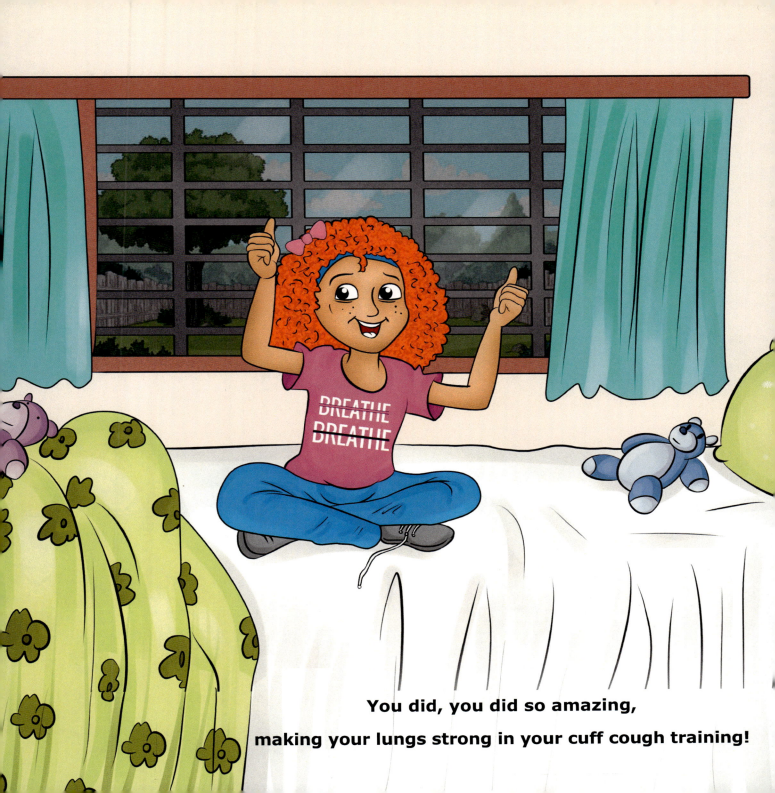

You did, you did so amazing,
making your lungs strong in your cuff cough training!

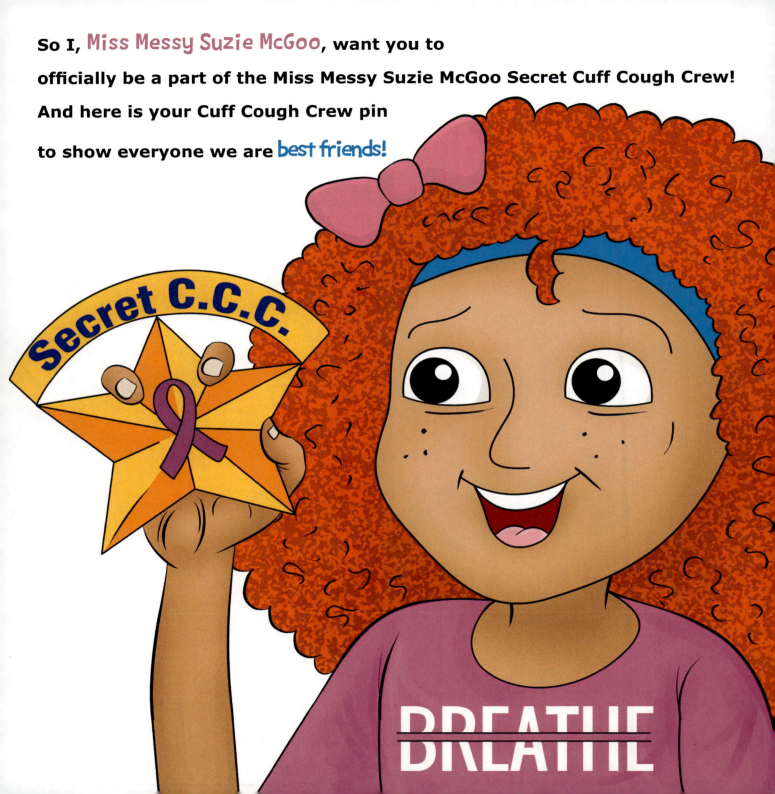

So I, Miss Messy Suzie McGoo, want you to officially be a part of the Miss Messy Suzie McGoo Secret Cuff Cough Crew! And here is your Cuff Cough Crew pin to show everyone we are best friends!

**Hippity dippity doppity diggity doo!
Y-a-a-a-y for me and you.**

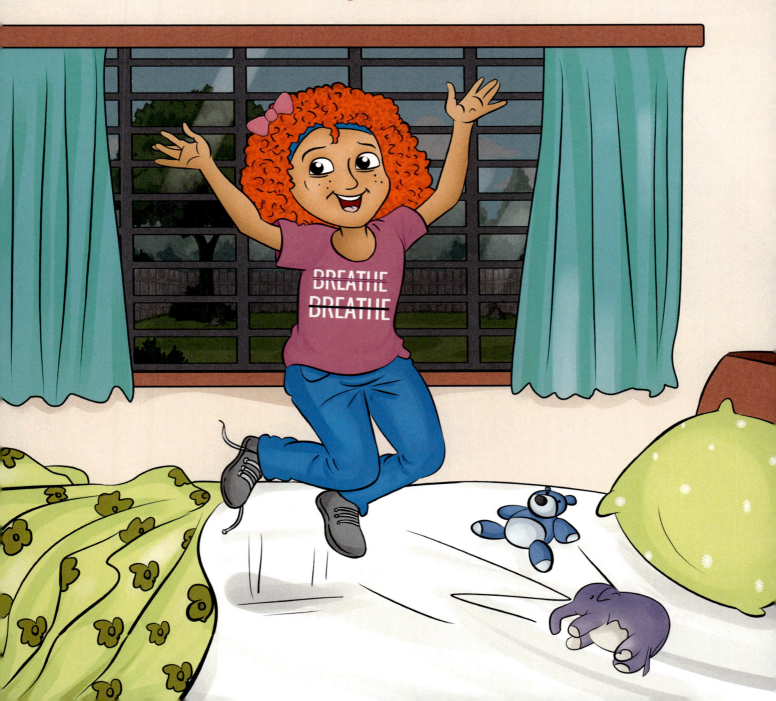

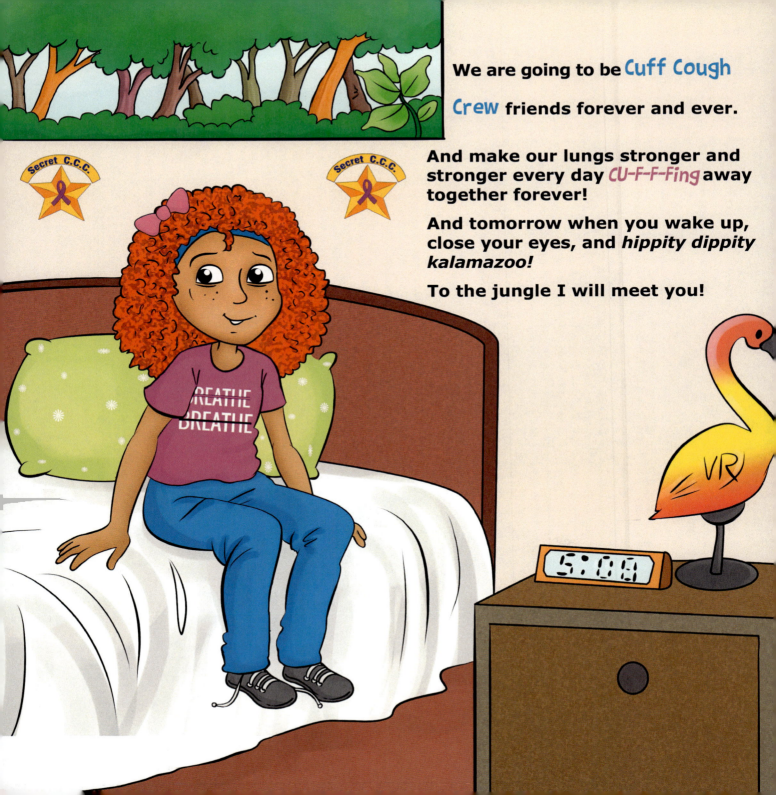

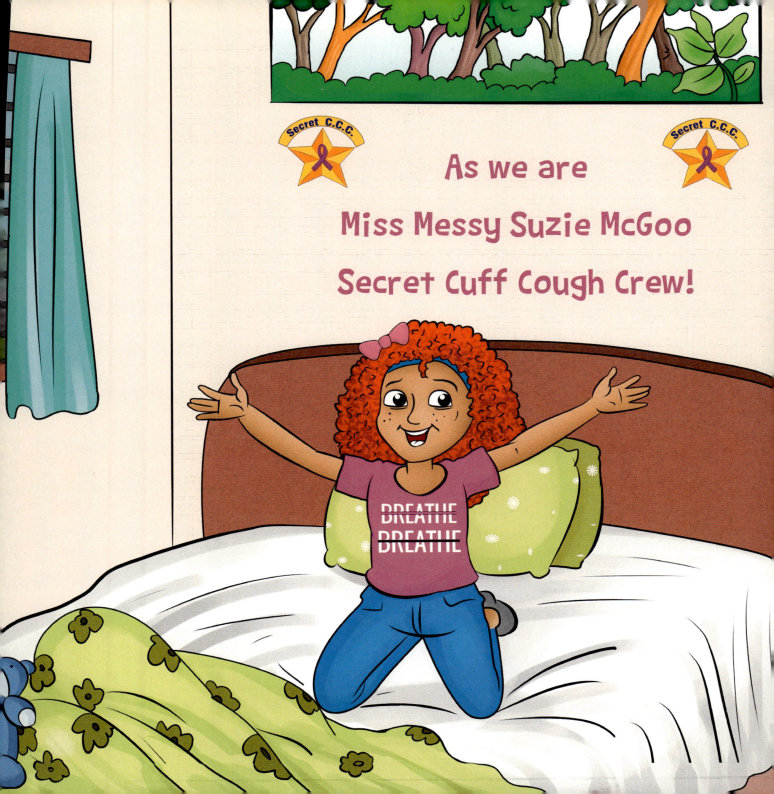

Author Bio Nicholas Kelly:

Nicholas Kelly's approach to life is filled with compassion, artistry, knowledge and a deep-rooted desire to do good in the world.

Diagnosed at three-months-old with cystic fibrosis by his mother, he never let his condition prevent him from pursuing a "normal" life. He worked hard, overcame obstacles, and thrived in all that he did, including earning a Bachelor's and Master's Degree from Bowling Green State University, after which he became, a dietitian.

In addition to his academic success, he is a poet, educator, dancer, and a decorated speaker. He draws from his personal experiences to inspire others to live to their full potential, use their strengths, remain positive, and advocate for themselves and others. He is an advocate for the CF community gaining recognition for his efforts in the media, national and local organizations, and patient centric speeches.

For more information about him, visit his website here:
www.NicholasKellyRD.com

For all things Suzie McGoo (updates, information, and merchandise) visit:
www.SuzieMcGoo.com

Author Bio for Maria Rohan:

Maria Rohan is a native of suburban Cleveland, OH. For the last decade, she has been a Cystic Fibrosis nurse. She has experienced firsthand the highs and lows of the disease and understands the impact it has on her patients' lives.

In addition to her direct patient care, Maria, a gifted writer, has been published for her work in Autism and child/adult trauma. Her passion and dedication extends beyond the clinical setting. She is a special needs basketball coach and an advocate for a kinder, more inclusive world that has compassion and a willingness to see life through a child's eyes.

Made in the USA
Las Vegas, NV
30 November 2021